Paleo Drinks

Delicious and Easy Paleo Drink

Recipes for Natural Weight Loss

and

A Healthy Lifestyle

By Elena Garcia

Copyright Elena Garcia © 2019

Disclaimer

A physician has not written the information in this book. It is advisable that you visit a qualified dietician so that you can obtain a highly personalized treatment for your case, especially if you want to lose weight effectively. This book is for informational and educational purposes only and is not intended for medical purposes. Please consult your physician before making any drastic changes to your diet.

All information in this book has been carefully researched and checked for factual accuracy. However, the author and publishers make no warranty, expressed or implied, that the information contained herein is appropriate for every individual, situation or purpose, and assume no responsibility for errors or omission. The reader assumes the risk and full responsibility for all actions and the author will not be held liable for any loss or damage, whether consequential, incidental, and special or otherwise, that may result from the information presented in this publication.

Contents

Introduction

Thank You for purchasing this book. It means you are very serious about your health and wellbeing.

Whether your goal it to lose weight, enjoy more energy or learn a few delicious healing recipes- you have come to the right place.

You are probably thinking...what? Paleo Drinks? What kind of a recipe book am I getting myself into? Does it mean I will be making some meat smoothies or juicing bacon? How about some egg tea?

The answer is no. This book will help you enrich your diet with a myriad of natural super healthy detoxifying drinks that will make you look and feel amazing. You will get a practical understanding of the best paleo drink recipes that are full of vitamins and minerals so that you can enjoy unstoppable energy.

The truth is, most people don't focus enough on what they drink. And they skip this amazing opportunity of vibrant health through paleo friendly hydration.

In case you are new to the paleo diet, the following pages will give you the easiest to follow healthy and balanced paleo lifestyle blueprint that is very easy to understand. Then, we will dive into paleo drink recipes as this is what this guide is all about.

So even if you are new to a healthy lifestyle-no worries, we got you covered.

And if you are already enjoying the wellness benefits that transitioning to a paleo diet and life offers, I am sure that the recipes contained in this book, will help you take it to the next level.

My goal is to make it as simple and doable as possible by giving you all the information, inspiration and recipes you need to transform your body while enjoying the process.

So...first of all, what is a paleo diet? Some kind of a cult? Or maybe a fad?

Well, some people in the health community love creating cults around diets, that's for sure.

But we like to keep it as easy to understand and follow as possible. Then, our goal is to make it easy, doable and fun- especially for a busy person. Eating a paleo diet means- eating foods that can be hunted or gathered while excluding processed foods.

And so, a paleo eater chooses:
-organic meat
-fresh fish and seafood
-organic eggs
-veggies
-fruits
-nuts & seeds
-herbs and spices (yes, they are paleo too!)

There is no dairy on a paleo diet. Instead of butter, it's recommended to use natural oils such as coconut oil or avocado oil. Milk is also off a paleo diet. Luckily, coconut milk and all kinds of nut milks are allowed. We are talking creamy cashew milk, aromatic coconut milk, delicious hazelnut milk. There are so many options out there!

To keep it simple – we just want to eat a natural, balanced diet and get rid of or reduce all processed foods.
Some people go paleo full time. Some do it part time. The truth is, even if you eat this way about 80% of time, you are good to go.

In this day and age, it's hard to keep a perfect diet.
But, creating vibrant health is all about balance, progress and healthy choices.

Most Paleo Diet beginners I talk to, think that going paleo is all about eating lots of meat and that's it.

Huge mistake. Our Paleolithic ancestors were also gatherers. So, aside from eating meat, they would also eat veggies, fruits, nuts and seeds. Oh, and herbs...

Nothing is every black and white. Balance is the key. That is how vibrant health is created.
Add to it relaxation, mindfulness, kindness and...some paleo drinks, which is what this recipe book is all about.

You see, even the healthiest paleo diet is doomed to fail if we forget about proper hydration.
Imagine our ancestors...I wonder...did they run on coffee all day? Drinking coffee and eating meat all day.

Does that sound reasonable?
Of course not. And you don't need to be an expert in nutrition to admit that.

I know I am exaggerating here. But, unfortunately, most people rely too much on coffee and forget about other drink alternatives.
That leads to dehydration. When you are dehydrated it's hard to focus, think clearly, feel motivated or even eat healthy.

It's very easy to misinterpret the feeling of dehydration as "I am feeling hungry again".

Now, it's time to re-connect with our Paleolithic ancestors and dive deep into a healthy, balanced lifestyle by giving yourself the optimal hydration we deserve.

That is why I decided to write this book. I want you to dive into my best paleo drink recipes that include smoothies, juices and teas.
It's time to nourish your body with a myriad of nutrients and healing recipes. Most people overlook the simple superfoods, herbs, fruits and

veggies that can be turned into natural and paleo friendly concoctions to help you stay energized.

This book is divided into 4 parts. The first part includes delicious paleo smoothies, including both naturally sweet smoothies as well as super tasty veggie smoothies. Many veggie smoothies can be turned into comforting soups, and you can even add in some meat or fish leftovers.

The second part is all about paleo juices, and the third part will help you discover the best of paleo friendly herbs, teas and infusions.
The fourth part is optional as it includes a mini paleo "crash course" to help you understand how this diet works.

Healthy eating is very easy when you commit to becoming resourceful. And it is my ultimate passion and mission. Through this book, I want to inspire you to start adding more delicious and nutritious paleo drinks to your diet.

To your health,
Enjoy!

About the Recipes-Measurements Used in the Recipes

The cup measurement I use is the American Cup measurement.

I also use it for dry ingredients. If you are new to it, let me help you:

If you don't have American Cup measures, just use a metric or imperial liquid measuring jug and fill your jug with your ingredient to the corresponding level. Here's how to go about it:

1 American Cup= 250ml= 8 fl.oz.

For example:

If a recipe calls for 1 cup of almonds, simply place your almonds into your measuring jug until it reaches the 250 ml/8oz mark.

I hope you found it helpful. I know that different countries use different measurements and I wanted to make things simple for you. I have also noticed that very often those who are used to American Cup measurements complain about metric measurements and vice versa. However, if you apply what I have just explained, you will find it easy to use both.

Part 1 Paleo Smoothie Recipes

Paleo smoothies are tasty, easy and quick to prepare even on a busy schedule. They can be used as a quick snack or breakfast. These smoothies are great for weight loss being full of fiber, vitamins and minerals. Some people find them useful for fasting or as a meal replacement.

You can play around with many of the ingredients and come up with your own favorites. You can leave things out or add some new ones so that you create the taste you love. That's what I love about them, they are so changeable but still so tasty and nutritious. Change things up and try something new. Have fun, be creative!

Note: be sure to wash all the fruits and veggies before turning them into smoothies.

Recipe #1 Banana Breakfast

This banana smoothie is perfect for breakfast and incorporates spirulina and kale, helping you to get in some extra nutrients in this morning smoothie. It is an energy boost that will keep you feeling full. You will get fiber, nutrients, and good, paleo friendly carbs in one glass!

Spirulina is an excellent superfood supplement to add to many foods or drinks to assist in weight loss.

Serves 1-2

Ingredients:

- 1 green apple, peeled
- 1 banana, peeled
- 1 tablespoon Spirulina
- ½ cup kale, peeled
- 1 cup coconut milk
- A few ice cubes

Instructions:

1. Place all the above ingredients in your blender.
2. Blend well.
3. Serve and enjoy!

Recipe #2 Berry Blaster

I love coconut water in my smoothie recipes because it is super hydrating and it has a wonderful flavor. When people get dehydrated one of the first signs is the feeling of hunger.

So, the good news is- by keeping yourself hydrated you will prevent unhealthy snack cravings.

Serves: 2

Ingredients:

- 1.5 cup of coconut water
- 1 cup blueberries, 1 cup of blackberries, 1 cup of raspberries (fresh)
- 1.5 cup spinach
- 2 tablespoons raw organic honey
- ¾ cup ice

Instructions:

1. Put all ingredients in a blender.
2. Pulse to desired consistency.
3. Enjoy!

Recipe #3 Paleo Hunger Hunter Smoothie

Avocados are full of healthy fats and nutrients. One half contains six grams of fiber. They contain protein, potassium and many vitamins. They keep my stomach full for hours. They are a super fruit. Not to mention they will add a lot of creaminess to any smoothie.

Egg yolks are a great addition to any smoothie on the paleo plan. Make sure they are organic and free-range or pasture raised. The yolks contain protein and omega 3s. They will fill you up and smash your hunger induced cravings.

Serves: 1

Ingredients:

- 1 avocado, peeled and pitted
- 1 large banana
- 2 cups of coconut or almond milk
- A cup of ice
- ¾ cup of kale
- ¾ cup of fresh spinach
- 2 egg yolks, organic

Instructions:

1. In a blender, add all the above ingredients except for the ice. Blend well.
2. Add ice and pulse until smooth.
3. Enjoy!

Recipe #4 Veggie Medley

Vegetables are an essential part of weight loss because they contain all of the vitamins our bodies require to run optimally.

Unfortunately, most people struggle with putting the veggies together. Not everyone enjoys a big bowl of salad with their meals. That is why paleo smoothies are an amazing solution. You can blend the veggies with some fruits and make sure you easily get all your healthy greens in, without even thinking about it.

Serves: 2-3

Ingredients:

- 2 handfuls of kale, chopped
- 2 stalks celery, chopped
- 1 cucumber, peeled and chopped
- 1 zucchini, peeled and chopped
- 1 lemon, peeled
- 1 big banana, peeled and chopped
- 2 cups almond milk, or any other paleo nut milk of your choice

Instructions:

1. Blend all and pulse in ice.
2. Enjoy!

Recipe #5 Easy Snack Smoothie

This smoothie will fill you up and you will not feel engorged or weighed down. It's just perfect when you feel like snacking. Why not drink this delicious smoothie instead?

Cranberries are high in vitamin C, among many other antioxidants. They help the body's conversion of glucose to energy.

Serves: 2

Ingredients:

- 2 teaspoons melted coconut oil
- 2 organic free-range egg yolks
- Handful of spinach
- 1 banana, peeled
- ½ cup cranberries
- 1 cup coconut water
- 1 cup coconut milk

Instructions:

1. Blend all and pulse in ice.
2. Enjoy!

Recipe #6 Healing Energy in a Glass

Feeling fatigued? You don't need another coffee. You already know that too much coffee can make you feel anxious...Try this smoothie instead as it will help you stay energized naturally.

Pepitas/pumpkin seeds are paleo-friendly and are great for weight loss. They contain quite a bit of zinc, which is important because it helps us produce testosterone to burn fat and build muscle. They also have magnesium and iron. Instant energy boost!

Serves: 3

Ingredients:

- ½ cup broccoli florets, chopped
- 1 cup spinach
- 1 egg yolk
- 1 tablespoon almond butter
- 1 tablespoon coconut oil
- Handful of pepitas
- 1 cucumber, peeled and chopped
- 1 ½ cup coconut water
- A few ice cubes

Instructions:

1. Blend all the above ingredients together in a blender except ice.
2. When well blended add the half cup ice and pulse.
3. Enjoy!

Recipe #7 Mental Energy Smoothie

Blueberries have been shown to improve brain function and motor skills. The recommendation is 1 cup/day. Avocado helps to lower blood pressure and allows for healthy blood flow; both of which affect brain function positively.

This smoothie is perfect if you need to study, work or concentrate for long periods of time.

Serves: 2

Ingredients:

- 1 cup blueberries, fresh
- 1 avocado, peeled and pitted
- 1 cup of almond or cashew milk
- 1/2 cup baby spinach

Instructions:

1. Place all the above ingredients in a blender, mix well and enjoy!

Recipe #8 Berry Antioxidant Weight Loss Smoothie

Blackberries contain more antioxidants than all of the other fruits on the Paleo plan. They are also rich in fiber content to help you stay full for hours, without feeling hungry.

Serves: 3-4

Ingredients:

- 1 cup of blueberries, fresh
- 1 cup blackberries, fresh
- 1 cup raspberries, fresh
- 2 cups almond milk
- ½ large banana, peeled
- Handful of greens of your choice

Instructions:

1. Blend all.
2. Serve and Enjoy!

Recipe #9 Mango Green Madness

This simple recipe combines the sweetness of mangos with the healing, alkalizing properties of spinach. Raw honey helps maintain a healthy immune system.

Serves: 2

Ingredients:

- 1 mango, peeled and sliced
- ½ banana, peeled
- 1 cup spinach
- 1 tablespoon raw honey
- A few ice cubes (optional)

Instructions:

1. Add all the above ingredients in a blender and blend well.
2. Pour and enjoy!

Recipe #10 Sweet Date Healing

This is one smoothie that I turn to whenever I am craving sweets. The cinnamon in this smoothie helps to regulate blood sugar and insulin levels in the body. And it tastes so delicious you crave more and more of it.

Go for it, it's all guilt free.

Serves: 1-2

Ingredients:

- 1/3 cup Medjool dates, pitted
- 1/2 cup ice
- 1 cup of almond or any other nut milk of your choice
- ½ avocado (peeled and pitted)
- 1 teaspoon of cinnamon powder
- Optional: 1 teaspoon melted coconut oil

Instructions:

1. Place all the above ingredients into the blender and mix/blend well.

Recipe 11 Vegetable Desire

After I had been eating a healthy, balanced paleo diet for a few months, I craved raw veggies constantly. That is why I came up with this simple veggie smoothie recipe, to make sure I get my daily portions of minerals and vitamins to look and feel amazing.

Serves: 2

Ingredients:

- 1 cup collard greens, Swiss chard, spinach mix
- 2 celery stalks, chopped
- ½ cup broccoli florets, chopped
- 1 cucumber, peeled and chopped
- 1 handful dandelion greens
- 2 Medjool dates
- 1 cup coconut water
- ½ c. ice

Instructions:

1. Place all the listed ingredients except for ice in a blender and mix/blend well.
2. Pulse in some ice.
3. Pour and enjoy.

Recipe #12 Simple Cream Smoothie

This is an amazing smoothie recipe if you are craving something sweet and creamy.

Serves: 1

Ingredients:

- 1 avocado (peeled and pitted)
- 1 small banana, peeled
- 1 tablespoon chia seeds
- 1 teaspoon cinnamon powder
- 1 teaspoon cocoa
- 1 cup coconut milk

Instructions:

1. Blend all except the ice for as long as possible.
2. Pulse in ice or skip the ice and freeze for ½ hour.
3. Enjoy!

Recipe #13 Mango Protein Smoothie

This smoothie is very high in protein and good fats which makes it an excellent breakfast smoothie as it will help you stay full till lunch.

Serves: 2

Ingredients:

- 1 frozen mango, chopped
- 3 tablespoons-soaked almonds
- 1 tablespoon powdered chia seeds
- 1.5 cup almond milk
- 1 cup spinach
- Half avocado, peeled, pitted
- Handful of blueberries

Instructions:

1. Blend all in a blender.
2. Enjoy the fruit of your labor!

Recipe #14 Guava Smoothie

Ginger and papaya are an amazing digestive mix. We are also getting in some greens to stay energized and guava to make it taste delicious.

Serves: 2

Ingredients:

- 1/2 cup of guava, chopped
- 1/2 cups spinach
- ½ lemon, peeled
- 1 teaspoon grated ginger
- ½ cup papaya, chopped
- 1 cup coconut water
- Ice, as needed

Instructions:

1. Place all the above ingredients in a blender. Carefully mix to attain the desired consistency.
2. Pulse in ice.
3. Enjoy!

Recipe #15 Cucumber Hydrating Green Smoothie

Cucumber is ultra-refreshing and full of healthy alkaline minerals such as magnesium.

Cilantro naturally works as a diuretic for the body.

This smoothie can also be served as a soup (warm or chilled).

If you want to serve it as a soup, I recommend you add in some hard-boiled eggs or smoked salmon. It really tastes delicious.

Enjoy!

Serves: 1

Ingredients:

- 2 cucumbers, peeled
- 1 celery stalk
- 1 avocado (peeled and pitted)
- Handful of cilantro
- 1 cup filtered water
- Pinch of Himalaya salt
- Pinch of black pepper
- Juice of half a lemon to taste

Instructions:

1. Blend all and refresh!

Recipe #16 Paleo Zucchini Zip

Zucchini is a wonderful option to be considered for the aim of weight loss. It contains few calories and is packed with vitamins and flavonoids. You can eat a ton of it without eating a bunch of calories. While, on its own, it may seem a bit boring, when blended with fruits and spices it really tastes amazing!

Serves: 1-2

Ingredients:

- 1 zucchini
- ½ green apple
- ¼ teaspoon cinnamon
- 1 cup spinach
- 1 cup coconut water
- ½ cup ice

Instructions:

1. Blend all ingredients.
2. Pulse ice and enjoy!

Recipe #17 Watermelon Dream

Watermelon is one of the most hydrating fruits and is also is an excellent fruit for weight loss.

Aside from being low in calories it is packed with nutrients. This recipe is perfect if you are working out. Watermelon is rich in the amino acid called citrulline and is useful in muscle recovery. Drink to your health!

Oh and we are sneaking in some greens too...

Serves: 2

Ingredients:

- 1 cup chopped watermelon
- 1 cup strawberries (fresh or frozen)
- A few broccoli florets
- ½ cup spinach
- 1 cup coconut water
- 1 teaspoon maca powder
- ½ cup ice (you can omit if using frozen berries)

Instructions:

1. Put all in a blender and mix to desired consistency.
2. Enjoy!

Recipe #18 Mediterranean Gazpacho Smoothness

Gazpacho is a traditional Spanish vegetable smoothie-like soup. It can be served both as a soup as well as a smoothie. It's one of my favorite lunch-time Paleo smoothies. Not only can it fill your stomach for hours and give you the necessary energy and healthy fats you need (olive oil), but also tastes out of this earth. If you decide to serve this recipe as a soup, my suggestion is to add in some ham, fried bacon or hard-boiled eggs for protein. You can also add in some chopped veggies of your choice, or any meat leftovers. Perfect meal for a busy schedule!

Serves: 2

Ingredients:

- 2 tablespoons green onion, sliced
- 2 tablespoons white ground pepper, chopped
- 2 tablespoon fresh lemon juice
- A handful of chopped celery
- ½ cup cucumber, peeled and chopped
- ¼ cup carrot, peeled and chopped
- 1 ½ cups peeled, diced and seeded tomatoes
- ½ cup almond, dairy free yogurt (you can also use coconut yoghurt)
- Half cup water, filtered
- 1 teaspoon ground black pepper
- 1 tablespoon extra-virgin olive oil

- 1 small clove of garlic
- Himalaya salt to taste
- 8 fresh basil leaves to garnish

Instructions:

1. Put all ingredients except basil leaves in blender and mix well.
2. If needed, add some more water and blend again.
3. Allow the gazpacho to cool.
4. Serve chilled in a bowl, decorated with basil leaves. Enjoy!
5.

Recipe #19 Celery Citrus Snack

This hydrating and refreshing smoothie is one of my favorites for warm weather. It's super hydrating and full of vital nutrients. The mint and citrus twist add an interesting flavor combination to the same vegetables that are used in most Paleo smoothies.

Mint is great for weight loss. Something about the taste suppresses appetite. Throw it in a smoothie and you will have added appetite suppression.

Serves: 1

Ingredients:

- 2 celery stalks
- 1 small cucumber, peeled and chopped
- Handful of spinach
- ½ lemon peeled
- 1 cup coconut milk
- ½ cup ice
- 3 mint leaves

Instructions:

1. Place the above ingredients in your blender and process until smooth.
2. Enjoy!

Recipe #20 Kale Green Powder Cup

Kale is a fabulous weight loss food because not only is it high in fiber to clean you out and help you feel full, it is packed with phytonutrients, tons of vitamins and minerals.

It is a super food and a sure-fire way to make sure you get a lot of it into your system every day is by supplementing what you eat with what you drink.

Serves: 1

Ingredients:

- 1 cup kale leaves
- 1 teaspoon spirulina powder
- 1 cup cashew milk (it tastes very creamy, however you can use any other nut milk)
- Half lemon, peeled
- 1 tablespoon coconut oil
- 1 green apple

Instructions:

1. Mix all in a blender.
2. Pour into your cup and enjoy!

Recipe #21 Delicious Baobab Smoothie

Baobab is rich in antioxidants, vitamin C, and potassium as well as digestive enzymes and probiotics. It also optimizes the absorption of iron. And of course, thanks to fiber, it helps you lose weight, and then keep it off. Tahini makes this smoothie super nutritious - sesame seeds provide the body with valuable nutrients, are a source of protein, magnesium, vitamin B12, healthy fat, calcium required for blood vessels, carbohydrates, amino acids, antioxidants (sesamol and sesamolin) – all this causes human cells to age more slowly. This smoothie is a perfect meal replacement and with its natural protein and healthy fats, it will help you feel full for hours.

Serves: 1-2

Ingredients:

- ½ teaspoon baobab fruit powder
- ½ teaspoon yacon powder / lucuma
- 1 cup fresh blueberries
- 1 cup almond milk
- Juice of 2 lemons
- 1/3 avocado
- 1 tablespoon of Tahini
- Optional: maple syrup, a few dates or stevia to sweeten, if needed

Instructions:

1. Using a blender, mix all the above ingredients together.
2. Enjoy!

Recipe #22 Choco Power Brain Smoothie

Cocoa has plenty antioxidants like the flavonoids and procyanidins (good agents for anti-ageing). It regenerates the body after exercise, both physically and mentally. It also significantly improves the functioning of the brain and memory.

Personally, I love this smoothie as a healthy, guilt-free treat.

At the same time, it's one of my favorite "power brain" smoothies for long writing sessions.

Serves: 1-2

Ingredients:

- 1 cup raw almond milk (without sugar)
- 6 pitted Medjool dates
- 1 small banana
- 3 tablespoons organic cocoa powder or few organic, paleo-friendly dark chocolate cubes (70%-90% is the best)
- 1 teaspoon melted coconut oil
- 1 teaspoon maca powder
- 1 teaspoon cinnamon powder
- 1 teaspoon chia seed powder (or chia seeds)

Instructions:

1. Put the almond milk, the dates and cocoa/chocolate in a blender first. Mix well. Add the banana, and blend again until everything is perfectly smooth.

2. Serve.

3. You may want to add or subtract from the cocoa, just adjust it to your own taste.

4. Enjoy!

Recipe #23 The Smashing Pumpkin

Frozen blueberries, ground cloves and fresh ginger will give this smoothie a very fresh, unique and enticing taste. I fell in love with it so many years ago! Pumpkin makes this smoothie full of good carbs that will help you stay energized for hours. You can also serve this smoothie as a thick, cold soup, or add in some nuts and seeds and serve it as a delicious, paleo smoothie bowl.

Serves: 1

Ingredients:

- 1 cup unsweetened almond or coconut milk
- ½ cup frozen blueberries
- A handful of cashew nuts
- ¼ teaspoon fresh ginger
- a teaspoon of ground cloves
- ½ cup smashed pumpkin

Instructions:

1. Put all ingredients in a blender and mix well.
2. Add ginger
3. Enjoy!

Recipe #24 Greens Sneaker

This smoothie is perfect for people who don't really like the idea of eating green salads.

I get that. I know that veggies and greens can get boring.

That is why, this recipe is just perfect, as you can easily get 2 cups of greens without even trying.

Serves: 2

Ingredients:

- 2 cups kale, fresh
- 2 cups coconut milk
- 1/2 cup pineapple, chopped
- 1 big kiwi, peeled
- 1 lime, peeled
- 1 teaspoon cinnamon powder
- A few fresh dates, pitted

Instructions:

1. Place all the other ingredients in a blender.
2. Blend and enjoy with ice cubes.

Recipe #25 Berry Best

This smoothie is a wonder in itself. It combines natural fiber and vitamin C from fresh fruits with an immune system boosting properties of honey.

To your health!

Serves: 3

Ingredients:

- 1 cup of coconut water
- 1 cup of blackberry
- 1 cup of raspberry
- 1 teaspoon chlorella powder
- A dash of honey
- Ice cubes

Instructions:

1. Blend all the ingredients in a food processor.
2. Pour in a tall glass, chill out the smoothie with ice cubes.

Recipe #26 Watermelon Berry Dream

Guava with watermelon and berries is a killer combination and it is a treat to Paleo eaters. Other than being super delicious and taste buds friendly, ingredients used in this smoothie also promote weight loss, as guava and watermelon provide the essential amount of fiber and the huge water content in watermelon helps keep the stomach full for a longer time, thereby curbing food cravings.

Serves: 2-3

Ingredients:

- 1 cup of watermelon, cubed, seeded and chilled
- Half cup strawberries
- Half cup blueberries
- 1.5 cup water, filtered
- ½ cup guava, chopped
- Ice cubes (optional)

Instructions:

1. Blend until thoroughly combined and smooth.
2. Toss in some ice cubes and enjoy.

Recipe #27 Papaya Weight Loss Surprise

Papaya is one of the best fruits to have while trying to reduce weight. It can also effectively help reduce bloating and other digestive problems. It combines really well with coconut oil and cinnamon powder, to help you reduce sugar cravings

Serves: 1-2

Ingredients:

- 1 small papaya, peeled, seeded and cubed
- 2 big carrots, peeled and chopped
- 1 cup coconut milk
- 1 tablespoon coconut oil
- 1 teaspoon cinnamon powder

Instructions:

1. Blend until smooth.
2. Toss in a few ice cubes and serve chilled.
3. Enjoy!

Recipe #28 Creamy Peach

This creamy smoothie is awesome for hot summer days. It's full of superfoods too. For example, maca powder helps re-balance hormones and Ashwagandha is an ancient Ayurvedic herb that helps sooth anxiety.

To learn more about this herb, I warmly invite you to read by book: "ASHWAGANDHA: The Miraculous Herb! Holistic Solutions & Proven Healing Recipes for Health, Beauty, Weight Loss & Hormone Balance".

For now, Ashwagandha is just a guest in this recipe, not the main hero.

Serves: 1-2

Ingredients:

- 1 cup coconut milk
- Half cup fennel tea, cooled down
- 1 peach, peeled and pitted
- 1 banana, peeled and pitted
- Half teaspoon maca powder
- Half teaspoon Ashwagandha powder
- 1 inch ginger, peeled
- 1 teaspoon lemon juice, fresh
- Some ice cubes

Instructions:

1. Place all the ingredients in a blender.
2. Blend until creamy and smooth.
3. Drop in ice cubes and enjoy the creamy smoothie chilled.

Recipe #29 Vitamin C Orange Smoothie

This recipe is just perfect if you are craving something sweet. It uses grapefruit and green tea. These are very helpful in weight loss and will help you stay energized. Green tea is also an amazing anti-oxidant.

Serves: 1-2

Ingredients:

- 1 whole orange, peeled and sliced
- 1 whole grapefruit, peeled and sliced
- 1 cup green tea, cooled down
- Half cup coconut water
- A handful of chopped pineapple

Instructions:

1. Place all the ingredients in a blender.
2. Process until smooth.
3. Drop a few ice cubes in the glass and serve right away.

Recipe #30 Creamy Spinach Beauty Smoothie

Spinach, avocado and lemon juice is a unique combination. It offers a miraculous mix of energy boosting minerals such as magnesium, iron and calcium. You can use this smoothie as a meal replacement or even serve it as a warm soup.

You can add in some nuts, seeds or meat leftovers.

Who said that paleo cooking has to be complicated? It's the easiest eating system there is.

Serves: 1

Ingredients:

- 1 cup of fresh spinach leaves
- 1 whole avocado, pitted, peeled and diced
- 1 teaspoon of fresh lemon juice
- 1 cup of cashew milk
- Black pepper and Himalaya salt to taste
- Fresh cilantro leaves to garnish
- Optional: 2 small chili flakes if you like it spicy

Instructions:

1. Blend all the ingredients until smooth.
2. Serve as it is or chilled with ice cubes.
3. Enjoy!

Recipe 31 Cherish Celery

This smoothie is full of the essential nutrients and vitamins like vitamin A, potassium, vitamin K2 and Vitamin B 6.

Coconut milk makes it very creamy and refreshing. It's also a perfect opportunity to add in some greens.

Serves: 1-2

Ingredients:

- ½ cup fresh cherries, pitted
- ½ cup of celery head
- A handful of spinach leaves, washed
- 2 tablespoons fresh mint leaves, one to add in to the smoothie, and one to garnish
- 1 cup of chilled coconut milk

Instructions:

1. Place all the ingredients and 1 tablespoon of fresh mint leaves in a blender.
2. Process until smooth.
3. Serve chilled with ice cubes and fresh mint leaves.
4. Enjoy!

Recipe #32 Healthy Skin Smoothie

This smoothie combines the beta carotene of carrots and tomatoes. Drink this smoothie on a regular basis and you will have a healthy-looking skin. Turmeric and ginger add to anti-inflammatory properties. Grapefruit is full of Vitamin C and natural anti-oxidants. One simple smoothie that combines so many superfoods, and all of them are easily accessible.

Plus, it tastes delicious and is very inexpensive to make.

Serves: 1-2

Ingredients:

- 1 cup of tomato, chopped and peeled
- ½ teaspoon of lemon juice
- 2 carrots
- 1 grapefruit, peeled
- 1 cup of water, filtered

Instructions:

1. Blend all the ingredients.
2. Serve the refreshing smoothie chilled.

Recipe #33 Simple Nutty Paleo Protein Smoothie

This smoothie combines natural, plant-based protein with digestive and weight loss properties of fresh apples. Paleo is not only about eating meat. It's also recommended to get some plant-based protein and eat some nuts and seeds. Healthy eating is all about balance and this is exactly what we are trying to inspire though this book.

Serves: 1-2

Ingredients:

- 2 green apples, peeled, chopped and de-seeded
- A handful of walnuts, soaked for a few hours
- A handful of hazelnuts, soaked for a few hours
- 1 cup hazelnut milk
- 1 teaspoon nutmeg powder
- 1 teaspoon cinnamon powder

Instructions:

1. Blend all the ingredients.
2. Serve and enjoy.

Recipe #34 Creamy Ginger Smoothie

Ginger is a very accessible superfood that very often gets overlooked.

The best way to use it is to add an inch or two to your smoothies.

Ginger adds to anti-inflammatory properties of your smoothies and it really tastes amazing.

Enjoy!

Serves: 1

Ingredients:

- 1 apple, peeled
- 1 cup coconut milk
- 1 banana, peeled
- 1 inch ginger, peeled
- 1 peach, pitted
- Optional: 1 teaspoon moringa powder

Instructions:

1. Blend the apple and banana slices with coconut milk.
2. Add the peach and crushed ginger.
3. Drop in a few ice cubes, serve and enjoy.

Part 2 Juices

Is juicing Paleo? Absolutely! These juices have a high concentration of zinc, calcium, iron, magnesium, phosphors, potassium, vitamins A, K, C, and E. They have lots of micronutrients, phytochemicals, chlorophyll and fiber.

While juicing can be a bit of a hussle and time-consuming, it's really worth it.

A 1 cup of fresh juice a day, or every other day is an excellent goal to begin with.

Health benefits of using Juices include:

- You give your digestive system a rest
- You get more energy
- It's easier to juice a mountain of fresh foods and veggies than to eat them
- Great for weight loss- you give your body a myriad of vitamins and nutrients with literally no calories. Your body gets hydrated and energized in a natural way and so you no longer crave unhealthy foods or sugars.

Juicing vs Smoothies? What is the Difference?

You are probably wondering what is better for you. Juicing vs Smoothies? The answer is – both are amazing.

It all depends on your health goals and personal preferences.

Juicing is a great option for people who want to increase their intake of fresh veggies and fruits, but their digestive systems are too sensitive to handle massive amounts of fiber.

So, in this case juicing is great! With juicing, you can get benefits of awesome produce without suffering any stomach issues for your juicing efforts.

Juices are easy to digest and easy to assimilate form.

Blending, as the name suggest and as you have already seen in the last chapter of this book- blends. With blending, you create smoothies that help you enjoy the benefits of fruits and veggies along with their gut friendly fiber.

However, and this is a very big however, people who are watching their blood sugar, sometimes prefer blending to juicing because the fiber ensures a slow and steady absorption of sugar into your bloodstream. Luckily, it is also possible to focus on creating juicing that are lower in sugar and this is the main focus of this chapter. We want to focus on making it as healthy as possible!

The golden rule is- when juicing, focus on:

-all kinds of veggies and greens that can be juiced

-low sugar fruit (for example: lemons, limes, pomegranates, grapefruits)

-adding bits of other fruit, to taste, is OK.

You will fully understand how it works, after we have dived into the recipes.

Tips for getting started with Juicing:

- Prepare your Schedule: Make sure it's a good time for you to do a cleanse and will be able to stick with it. Going on a cruise or having your in-laws visit you would not be a good time to do it!
- Prepare your House: Clean out the fridge and pantry and be sure it's stocked with tons of fresh and frozen produce.
- Begin by adding a handful or so of organic baby spinach into your juices especially if you're new to green juices.
- Invest in a good juicer and prepare to spend some time in the kitchen. Juicing takes a lot of washing, cutting and clean-up.
- Prepare all your juices the night before and store them in air-tight containers for the following day. Making all the juices at once can save time in clean up and ensures you're ready with fresh juice whenever needed
- There are so many variations of Juicing, you can use the recipes and add or take away ingredients. Feel free to swap for your favorite ingredients, just make sure you're getting a good variety throughout the day.

The juicer I like to use is Omega Juicer. However, any other cold pressed juicer will do.

Make sure you wash all the ingredients before you proceed to your juicing rituals.

Now, back to the recipes!

Recipe #35 Cucumber Kale and Carrot Juice

Cucumber has 90% of water in them that plays an important role in breaking fat cells. Eating cucumber in plenty is wonderful since they are a natural procedure for weight loss.

While it's hard to eat a mountain of greens and cucumbers, it's easy to drink their juice and get all the vital nutrients in. Avocado oil offers good fat to help you absorb the minerals and vitamins from the juice.

Servings: 2

Ingredients:

- 2 big carrots, peeled and chopped
- 1 lemon, peeled
- 3 celery stalks, chopped
- A couple dashes of habanero hot sauce
- a handful of kale, chopped
- 2 big cucumbers, peeled and chopped
- a drizzle of avocado oil

Instructions:

1. Place through a juicer.
2. Juice.
3. Pour into a glass and add in a couple dashes of habanero hot sauce, if needed.

Recipe #36 Flavored Spinach Juice

While pure spinach juice can be a bit hardcore, this recipe is a bit different.

Add in some fresh apples and ginger and you will fall in love with green juice.

One green juice a day will keep the doctor away!

Serves: 2

Ingredients:

- 2 cups of fresh spinach
- 2 green apples, peeled and chopped
- 2-inch ginger, peeled
- 1 tablespoon melted coconut oil

Instructions:

1. Place all the ingredients through a juicer.
2. Extract the juice, pour it in a big glass.
3. Add in some melted coconut oil.
4. Stir well and enjoy.

Recipe #37 Watermelon Antioxidant Juice

Watermelon, ginger and healing greens is an excellent combination. It makes the juice taste nice and helps you get accustomed to juicing greens.

Servings: 2

Ingredients:

- 1 cup of watermelon, chopped
- 1 cup mixed greens of your choice (I like to throw in some spinach, arugula and mint)
- 2 inch of ginger, peeled

Instructions:

1. Juice all the ingredients using a juicer.
2. Serve in a glass.
3. Enjoy!

Recipe #38 Simple Apple Lemon Juice

Apples help maintain a healthy digestive system.

Oh and they make green juices taste great!

Servings: 2

Ingredients:

- 2 cups of kale, chopped
- 2 apples, peeled and chopped
- 1 lemon, peeled and halved
- 1 inch of ginger, peeled
- 1-inch turmeric, peeled

Instructions:

1. Place all the ingredients in a juicer.
2. Juice and serve in a glass.
3. Enjoy!

Recipe #39 Honeydew Melon Green Juice

This is a super hydrating juice that combines the healing power of veggies and fruits.

While a pure green juice may be a bit too much for a beginner, adding in some honeydew melon really takes it to a whole new level.

Servings: 2

Ingredients:

- 4 medium cucumbers, peeled and chopped
- 1 cup of honeydew melon
- 4 cup romaine lettuce

Instructions:

1. Place all the ingredients through a juicer.
2. Extract the juice.
3. Pour into a chilled glass and enjoy!

Recipe #40 Easy Green Juice

Red bell peppers are one of my favorite veggies to juice.

They are natural sweet and full of vitamins and minerals. They make any green juice taste amazing. Ginger adds to anti-inflammatory properties.

Servings: 2

Ingredients:

- 1 cup celery, chopped
- 3 red bell peppers, chopped
- 1 inch of ginger, peeled
- 2 slices of lime, to garnish
- Fresh ice cubes

Instructions:

1. Juice all the ingredients using a juicer.
2. Pour in a glass, add in some ice cubes.
3. Garnish with lime slices.
4. Serve and enjoy!

Recipe #41 Coconut Kale Concoction

Compared to other juicing recipes, this one is relatively simple and quick to make as it leverages the coconut water. Just perfect as a quick, energy boosting juice

Servings: 2

Ingredients:

- 1 cup kale, chopped
- 1 green apple, cut into smaller pieces
- 1 cup of coconut water
- 1 teaspoon cinnamon powder

Instructions:

1. Juice the kale and apple.
2. Pour into a glass and mix with 1 cup of coconut water.
3. Stir well, add in 1 teaspoon of cinnamon powder and stir again.

Recipe #42 Broccoli and Orange Juice

This juice is great for boosting your energy and stimulating weight loss.

It combines the healing and immune system boosting benefits of Vitamin C from oranges with the detoxifying properties of chlorophyll from the broccoli.

Servings: 2

Ingredients:

- 1 cup broccoli, chopped
- 4 oranges, peeled and cut into smaller pieces
- 1 lemon, peeled and cut into smaller pieces
- 1-½ cups of alkaline water

Instructions:

1. Place through a juicer.
2. Juice, and pour into a jar or a big glass and add in some water (you can skip this step if you like the intense taste of this juice)
3. Enjoy!

Recipe #43 Green Tea High Energy Juice

This recipe is similar to the last one, however it also uses green tea to help you boost your energy levels and burn fat. Ginger adds to anti-inflammatory properties.

Servings: 2

Ingredients:

- 3 oranges, peeled and cut into smaller pieces
- Half cup spinach leaves
- 1 inch ginger, peeled
- 1 cup green tea, cooled down

Instructions:

1. Juice the oranges, ginger and spinach.
2. Pour into a glass or a jar and add in some green tea.
3. Enjoy!

Recipe #44 A Beta Carotene Powerhouse

This juice is a fantastic combination of oranges, turmeric and carrots to help you have beautiful and healthy-looking skin while enjoying more energy without having to rely on caffeine.

Servings: 2

Ingredients:

- 6 carrots, peeled and chopped
- 2 oranges, peeled and cut into smaller pieces
- 1 lemon, peeled and cut into smaller pieces
- 1 zucchini, peeled and cut into smaller pieces
- 2-inch turmeric, peeled
- A few ice cubes (optional)
- A dash of cinnamon powder (optional)

Instructions:

1. Juice all the ingredients.
2. Pour into a glass and add in some ice cubes and a dash of cinnamon powder.
3. Enjoy!

Recipe #45 A Restorative Antioxidant Juice

This juice is full of antioxidants and beta-carotene to help you have beautiful skin.

Servings: 2

Ingredients:

- 4 large Carrots, peeled and chopped
- 4 tomatoes, cut into smaller pieces
- 1 Garlic clove, peeled
- 1-inch ginger, peeled

Instructions:

1. Juice all the ingredients.
2. Pour into a glass and enjoy!

Recipe #46 Veggie Medley Juice

Enjoy the wonderful mixture full of ingredients that make you healthy. They also contain antioxidant and elements that will help your body to fight against diseases and help in weight loss.

Servings: 4

Ingredients:

- 6 medium carrots, peeled and cut into smaller pieces
- 1 beet (with greens), peeled
- 3 large tomatoes, cut into smaller pieces
- 1 to 2 large handfuls spinach
- 1/8 head cabbage, chopped
- 3 kale leaves
- 1 red bell pepper, chopped
- 1 large celery stalk, chopped
- ¼ yellow onion, chopped
- ½ clove garlic, peeled
- ½ bunch parsley (optional)

Instructions:

1. Juice all the ingredients.
2. Pour into a glass.
3. If needed, season with some Himalaya salt.
4. Enjoy!

Recipe #47 Cabbage and Coconut Juice

This recipe has plenty of antioxidants and is full of refreshing nutrients.

While pure green juice might be a bit too "hardcore" even for experienced juicing fanatics, it tastes amazing when mixed with other ingredients.

Servings: 1

Ingredients:

- ½ Cabbage, chopped
- ½ cup coconut water
- 4 green apples, chopped

Instructions:

1. Juice all the ingredients.
2. Pour into a glass and mix with some coconut water.
3. Enjoy!

Recipe #48 Mixed Green Juice

This recipe is great if you happen to have some arugula leaves leftovers and don't feel like going for another salad. And yes, arugula juice tastes amazing when mixed with other ingredients!

Servings: 2

Ingredients:

- 1 cup arugula leaves
- A few pineapples slices
- 1 orange, peeled and cut into smaller pieces
- 1 lemon, peeled and cut into smaller pieces

Instructions:

1. Place though a juicer.
2. Juice and pour into a glass or a small jar.
3. Enjoy!

Recipe #49 Tantalizing Green Juice

Once again, we are juicing arugula leaves while adding in some sweetness and vitamin C from Kiwis and anti-inflammatory benefits of ginger. Apple helps in digestion and lime adds even more of vitamin C and refreshing aroma.

Servings: 2

Ingredients:

- 1 cup arugula leaves
- 2 kiwis, peeled
- 1 green apple, cut into smaller pieces
- 1 lime, peeled and cut into smaller pieces
- 1-inch ginger, peeled

Instructions:

1. Place all the ingredients though a juicer.
2. Juice and enjoy!

Recipe #50 Healing Carrot Juice

Carrot juice tastes amazing and when combined with cucumber juice, it will help you stay hydrated and reduce unwanted sugar cravings for hours. Ashwagandha powder is optional here.
But it's a great choice to help you re-balance your energy levels while feeling more relaxed.

Servings: 2

Ingredients:

- 6 carrots, peeled and chopped
- 3 big cucumbers, peeled and chopped
- ¼ teaspoon Ashwagandha powder

Instructions:

1. Juice all the ingredients.
2. Pour into a glass and enjoy!

Recipe #51 Cucumber's Delight

Cucumber contains water that provides a good environment for hydration and therefore contributes to weight loss. Parsley leaves add in a ton of vitamins and nutrients such as Vitamin A, Vitamin C and Iron. Mint helps in digestion and brings an amazing aroma to the table.

Servings: 2

Ingredients:

- 2 large cucumbers, peeled and chopped
- A handful of fresh mint leaves
- A handful of fresh parsley leaves

Instructions:

1. Juice all the ingredients.
2. Pour into a glass or a small jar.
3. Enjoy!

Recipe #52 Turmeric Green Juice

Turmeric is full of polyphenols that help well in weight loss.

It's a great addition to your juices and creates a nice, spicy aroma that is very easy to get hooked on.

Servings: 2

Ingredients:

- 2 inch turmeric, peeled
- 2 inch ginger, peeled
- 2 oranges, peeled and cut into smaller pieces
- 1 lemon, peeled and cut into smaller pieces
- Half cup water, filtered

Instructions:

1. Juice all the ingredients.
2. Pour into a glass and mix with water.
3. Enjoy!

Recipe #53 Pineapple Lime Mint Juice

This recipe balances the energy and weight loss stimulating benefits of greens with the sweetness of pineapple.

Servings: 3-4
Ingredients:

- ½ cup kale, chopped
- 1 cup pineapple, chopped
- ¼ cup mint leaves, fresh
- 2 limes, peeled and chopped

Instructions:

1. Place through a juicer.
2. Juice and pour into a glass.
3. Enjoy!

Recipe #54 Orange Pomegranate Juice

With Orange Pomegranate, you are sure of enjoying juice that is full of antioxidants and nutrients that are good for weight loss.

Oh, and we are snaking in some greens too. Great way to make use of some salad leftovers.

Servings: 2

Ingredients:

- 1 cup pomegranate seeds
- 1 cup of mixed greens of your choice
- 2 oranges, peeled and cut into smaller pieces

Instructions:

1. Place through a juicer.
2. Pour into a glass and enjoy!

Recipe #55 Coconut Flavored Green Juice

The ingredients are rich in phytonutrients and antioxidants. The juice relaxes the body and makes it easy to lose extra pounds.

Servings: 2

Ingredients:

- 1 cup kale, chopped
- 2 tablespoons coconut oil
- 1 cup pineapple, chopped
- 1 green apple, chopped

Instructions:

1. Place all the ingredients through a juicer.
2. Juice and pour into a glass
3. Enjoy!

Part 3 Teas and Herbal Infusions

When you mention the word *detoxification*, you can't miss the benefits of tea.

Black and green teas have antioxidants in them, good for the detoxification process and alleviating the risks of chronic inflammation. Herbal tea contains infusions that comprise of spices and herbs and does not contain caffeine.

Tea is good for flushing out unwanted toxins from your body and has the capacity to cut down on the fat cells too.

You've probably heard of Chinese men and women living well past the 100-year mark. Most of them attribute their long life to drinking tea. They consume the tea on a daily basis and drink 2-3 times a day.

Tea helps to boost your energy as well. It's the caffeine that helps in increasing your energy and keeping you fit. You will have enough energy to last throughout a busy day. If you wake up feeling out of sorts, a refreshing cup of tea can chase the blues away and lighten your mood.

If you suffer from insomnia or have trouble sleeping, then herbal tea can help to solve the problem. By consuming chamomile tea on a regular basis, you can effectively eliminate the problem and fall asleep much more easily. Apart from chamomile, there are also other concoctions that you can brew and consume to fall asleep better.

We will look at these teas in the following recipes.

Recipe #56 Ginger and Turmeric Tea

This tea is great for getting rid of coughs and colds and will perform wonders for those looking to lose excess weight.

Serves: 1

Ingredients:

- 1 inch ginger, peeled
- 1 inch turmeric, peeled
- 1 cup water, boiling
- 1 Indian spice blend tea bag
- 1 teaspoon honey

Instructions:

1. Place all the tea ingredients (except honey) in a tea pot and pour over some boiling water.
2. Keep covered for 15 minutes.
3. Strain and serve warm (but not boiling) in a tea cup with 1 teaspoon of honey.

Note: If you are unable to find the Indian spice tea bags then you can prepare your own. To prepare the tea bag mix together tea leaves along with a couple of cloves, 1 black cardamom pod, 1 teaspoon black pepper corns, ½ inch cinnamon stick and a few green cardamom pods.

Recipe #57 Easy Chili Tea

This tea will help in cleansing your digestive tract while warming

you up and giving you a strong energy boost that will last for hours.

Serves: 2

Ingredients:

- 2 cups water, boiling.
- 2 green tea bags
- 2 red chili flakes
- A handful of fresh mint leaves
- 2 tablespoons honey

Instructions:

1. Place all the tea ingredients (except honey) in a tea pot and pour over 2 cups of boiling water.
2. Keep covered for 15 minutes.
3. Strain and serve warm (but not boiling) in a tea cup with 1 teaspoon of honey.

Recipe #58 Cumin and Caraway Tea

This tea is great for those women looking to obtain relief from period cramps.

Serves: 1-2

Ingredients:

- 2 cups water, boiling
- 1 black tea bag (optional, if you need an energy boost but you can skip it if you want to keep it 100% caffeine-free)
- 1 inch ginger, peeled
- 1 tablespoon cumin seeds
- 1 tablespoon caraway seeds
- 1 tablespoon coriander seeds
- 1 tablespoon fennel seeds
- 1 tablespoon honey, if needed

Instructions:

1. Place all the tea ingredients (except honey) in a tea pot and pour over 2 cups of boiling water.
2. Keep covered for 15 minutes.
3. Strain and serve warm (but not boiling) in a tea cup with 1 teaspoon of honey.

Recipe #59 Spicy Chai Tea

This tea is super tasty and creamy. It can be consumed on a regular basis and it's great to prevent colds too.

Serves: 1-2

Ingredients:

- 1 cup almond or coconut milk
- 1 Indian chai tea bag
- 2 inch turmeric, peeled
- 2 tablespoons honey

Instructions:

1. Boil almond milk using a saucepan
2. When boiling, add the tea bag and turmeric.
3. Simmer on low heat for 5 minutes.
4. Turn off the heat and keep covered for 15 minutes.
5. Pour into a tea cup and sweeten with honey if needed

In the absence of chai tea, make use of tea leaves mixed with cinnamon, cloves and cardamon Make it sweet and healthy by adding the almond milk.

Recipe #60 Ashwagandha Tea

This is a great tea for those looking to boost their sex drive. It is also good for those looking to increase their immunity.

Serves: 1-2

Ingredients:

- 1 tablespoon dried ashwagandha
- 2 cups water, boiling
- 1 fennel tea bag
- 1 green tea bag
- 1 tablespoon honey (optional)

Instructions:

1. Place all the tea ingredients (except honey) in a tea pot and pour over some boiling water.
2. Keep covered for 15 minutes.
3. Strain and serve warm (but not boiling) in a tea cup with 1 teaspoon of honey (if needed)

Recipe #61 Sleep Well Tea

This recipe will help you unwind after a busy day, sleep like a baby and wake up feeling energized.

Serves: 2

Ingredients

- 1 cup of water, boiling
- 1 lemongrass stalk
- 2 tablespoons chamomile tea
- A few tablespoons of coconut milk
- 1 tablespoon of coconut oil
- A dash of cinnamon powder to garnish

Instructions:

1. Place all the tea ingredients (except coconut milk and oil) in a tea pot and pour over some boiling water.
2. Keep covered for 15 minutes.
3. Strain.
4. Pour into a tea cup and add in the coconut milk and oil.
5. Stir well.
6. Sprinkle over some cinnamon powder, enjoy!

Bonus Recipe: Easy Mediterranean Tea

This tea can be made in 2 different ways:

1.You can choose to add in some green tea, if you need more energy, for example if you are using this tea in the morning.

2.You can choose to add in some Melissa tea, if you need to unwind, for example if you are using this tea in the evening and want to unwind and sleep well.

Rosemary and fennel are both miraculous herbs and will help you boost your immune system and fight off colds and flu.

Fennel is also great for weight loss as well as stimulating your lymphatic system.

Serves:2

Ingredients:

- 2 cups boiling water
- 1 tablespoon rosemary herb
- 1 tablespoon fennel seeds
- 1 teaspoon green tea, or Melissa tea (optional)

Instructions:

1. Place all the tea ingredients (except honey) in a tea pot and pour over some boiling water.
2. Keep covered for 15 minutes.
3. Strain and serve warm (but not boiling) in a tea cup with 1 teaspoon of honey (if needed)

Bonus Recipe: Lime Refresher Ice Tea

Blueberries are known for their anti-oxidant providing abilities and they are wonderfully sweet. Add the addition of spicy herb and a lime twist, and you have a hydrating drink that is fully paleo!

Ingredients

- 2 cups of blueberries
- 2 limes
- 1 medium bunch of fresh oregano
- 1 liter of water – filtered if liked

Instructions

1. Pour the water in to a suitable container or jug.
2. Wash the blueberries and limes.
3. Add the blueberries to the water, squashing a third of them on to a plate beforehand, and catching any juice to add too.
4. Juice one of the limes and add the juice to the water. Slice the other lime in to thin pieces.
5. Wash the oregano and give it a bit of a "squeeze" to start releasing some of it's flavor.
6. Add the herbs to the water and mix really well. Leave in the fridge for at least an hour before serving.

Final Words and Your Paleo Quick Start Guide

We hope you enjoyed the recipes and feel inspired to live a Paleo lifestyle. We are adding this short Paleo guide to help you on your health journey. Remember, it's not about being perfect. Even if you do Paleo "part time", but you listen to your body and focus on adding as many healthy foods as possible, you are good to go.

It's not about going hungry or getting too caught up in counting calories.

Paleo Lifestyle Made Easy

The Paleo diet is an approach to eating that originated a long time ago, during the Paleolithic era. This time frame started about 2.5 million years ago and ended around 10,000 years before our time. It avoids eating foods that only became part of the human diet after the agricultural revolution. The idea is that diseases like cancer and diabetes started around the same time that we began growing our own foods. The underlying principle is that the hunter-gatherers' diet is the reason they did not develop such diseases.

While we cannot be sure that their diet is what kept them healthy, there is enough research that concludes that foods banned from Paleo diets have little or no beneficial nutritional value. They have also been proven to interrupt normal hormonal balances, cause inflammation, and damage the lining of the gut. Eating Paleo will help to balance our bodies internally, protect the kidneys, protect the digestive tract from destructive proteins like gluten, and keep the liver and pancreas from having to work too hard.

Many names and titles have been given to this age-old eating program: the Paleolithic diet, Paleolithic nutrition, Paleo diet, Stone Age diet, caveman diet, and hunter-gatherer diet. Paleo Diet is an effort to go back to eating how we were biologically intended to eat. This method enables us to fuel our bodies properly so that they may function at their full genetic potential and start living healthier immediately. Foods that could be collected and consumed by hunting and gathering are what need to focus on. Primal eating at its best.

For me, I like to think of it as a Paleo perspective, not an actual diet. It could also be called a template. However you look at it, it is a lifestyle change. The goal is to eat like our ancestors did millions of years ago before the Agricultural Revolution.

Here are seven guidelines for Paleo nutrition that helped me to get a better idea of the principles involved in this primal nutritional practice.

1. **Increase protein intake.**

15% of the calories in most diets are from protein. When adhering to Paleo, that percentage must be much higher. It should be between 19-35 percent. A large amount of animal protein is required.

2. **Decrease carbohydrate intake and eat foods lower on the glycemic index.**

Most of the carbs will come from vegetables (and a few fruits). They should take up between 35-45 percent of your daily caloric intake. Most of the foods you will eat will be low on the glycemic index. They will not make your blood sugar spike because they are assimilated slowly.

3. Increase fiber consumption.

Paleos get their fiber from non-starchy vegetables. Vegetables such as these usually contain a fiber content around 30 percent higher than processed grain and about eight times higher than whole grain. Even fruits have more fiber than whole and refined grains.

4. Increase fat intake by eating more monounsaturated and polyunsaturated fats.

You need to do this in combination with a good balance of Omega-3 and Omega-6 fats. It is a common misconception that health is related to how *much* fat you eat, when the *type* of fat you eat affects your health more. Increase monounsaturated and Omega-3 fats and remove Trans and Omega-6 polyunsaturated fats.

5. Raise potassium while lowering sodium.

Paleolithic humans consumed foods that were unrefined and fresh. Potassium levels in fresh foods are between 5-10 percent higher than sodium levels. Potassium helps the heart, kidneys, and other organs function correctly. People who have low potassium levels are more susceptible to elevated blood pressure, stroke, and cardiovascular disease. Excessive sodium levels can also cause the same problems. Many modern diets contain two times as much sodium as potassium.

6. Eat more alkaline than acidic foods.

When we consume food, it has either an acid or alkaline effect on your body. Even on a Paleo diet, it is necessary to keep this in mind because meat and fish are both acid-forming foods. Alkaline-producing foods include most vegetables and fruits. Having an acidic system for a long time can lead to atrophy of the muscles and bone, elevated blood pressure, kidney stones, and can trigger things like asthma and allergies.

7. **Increase the intake of vitamins, phytochemicals, minerals, and antioxidants.**

Whole grains are a poor source of these things. The few minerals and vitamins that are actually in whole grains are not usually processed and absorbed properly by the body. They do not contain vitamin C, A, or B12. There truly is no substitute for grass-produced and free-range meat or organic vegetables and fruits.

What foods did the cavemen eat? What foods did they hunt, and what did they go out and gather? These are two key questions to keep in mind when deciding what to eat on the Paleo diet.

Basic categories of foods to consume when eating Paleo:

➤ Grass-produced meats
➤ Fish and seafood
➤ Eggs
➤ Fresh fruits and vegetables
➤ Seeds
➤ Healthful oils (olive, walnut, flaxseed, macadamia, avocado, or coconut)

The foods included on the Paleo diet are foods that our cave-dwelling ancestors would have access to on a regular basis.

Basic categories of what NOT to eat when eating Paleo:

- Cereals and grains
- Potatoes
- Legumes
- Sugars
- Processed foods
- Salt
- Dairy
- Refined vegetable oil

Some people do not understand exactly what a legume is. A legume is the seed pod of a plant that is edible. Examples of legumes are:

- Beans
- Peas
- Lentils
- Soy

Essentially, if a caveman could not have eaten it 10,000 years ago, you cannot eat it now. No consuming packaged foods at all. If it contains chemicals or ingredients that you cannot pronounce, then it is probably not Paleo.

Inflammation is the body's natural response to invaders. I already discussed this problem and how "leaky gut" will lead to weight gain. It may be more important to note that "leaky gut" will lead to major health issues because it causes chronic inflammation. Cancer, asthma, headaches, allergies, arthritis, auto-immune disorders, heart disease, diabetes, depression, Alzheimer's, and osteoporosis are all caused by chronic inflammation. The list goes on and on.

Why does inflammation cause so many problems? Inflammation is an immune system response. It is used by the body to battle intruders that are unidentified or already deemed harmful. Well, how could something good cause such a problem? Let me explain it this way. It is like leaving the heater turned up and the thermostat not working. It never turns off when the environment gets to a certain temperature. Yes, you wanted to warm up, but if it never turns off, it will get way too hot. It will negatively affect whatever is in the environment.

Converting to a Paleolithic nutritional lifestyle has allowed me to eat a diet that is void of inflammatory foods. Aside from healing "leaky gut," thus allowing the immune system to calm down, Paleo diets also reduce inflammation in many other ways. I have highlighted a few below:

➢ The diet is high in vitamin D. Vitamin D has been proven to aid in reducing inflammation.

➢ The diet is high in phytonutrients, many of which have anti-inflammatory effects.

➢ The immune system reacts to factors in the environment that it has been exposed to (pollen, bacteria, molds, etc.) with inflammation. The Paleo diet has the effect of making the immune system less prone to react to these factors and also makes it more effective because it is not over-loaded.

➤ The Paleo perspective adjusts the Omega-3/Omega-6 proportion to a beneficial ratio and makes it an effective agent in battling inflammatory illnesses. An Omega-3/6 imbalance can result from eating vegetable oils, grain products, and a deficiency of DHA and EPA from animal products.

Reading labels is a must-do for any Paleo dieter. For the most part, anything with a label is probably something you do not want to buy. If it does have a label, but you can't pronounce the ingredients, do not purchase it. Here are some things that I keep in mind when I grocery shop:

Best = Zero ingredients

Better = One ingredient

Ok = Two ingredients

Pushing my luck = Three ingredients

No way = Four+ ingredients

Key words to remember when shopping to stock a Paleo kitchen:
Organic, grass-fed, pasture-raised, wild-caught, free-range, and raw.

I had to replace everything in my pantry with new ingredients that I would be using in Paleo recipes. I had previewed these new recipes, and if you are anything like me, these ingredients sounded strange. They are staples of the Paleo kitchen and will benefit you in preparing many delicious Paleo meals and snacks. This a list of items that are usually used in Paleo recipes:

- **Blanched almond flour**

- **Coconut flour**

- **Almond meal**

- **Extra virgin coconut Oil**

- **Refined coconut oil**

- **Palm shortening**

- **Arrowroot powder/Tapioca starch**

- **Ground flax meal**

- **Coconut milk**

- **Creamed coconut**

- Unsweetened coconut flakes

- Unsweetened shredded coconut

- Nuts: Whole almonds, pecan halves, walnut halves, macadamia nuts, hazelnuts, pistachios, cashews, Brazil nuts

- Almond Butter

- Raw/natural cocoa powder

- Honey

- Raw maple syrup

- Leavening/Spices: Baking soda, cream of tartar, allspice, cinnamon, salt, cloves, cardamom, ground ginger, nutmeg, vanilla extract, vanilla bean, lemon juice

We Need Your Help

One more thing, before you go, could you please do us a quick favor?

It would be great if you could leave us a short review on Amazon.

Don't worry, it doesn't have to be long. One sentence is enough.

Let others know your favorite recipes and who you think this book can help.

Your opinion is very important.

Thank You once again for your support!

Join Our VIP Readers' Newsletter to Boost Your Wellbeing

Would you like to be notified about our new health and wellness books? How about receiving them at deeply discounted prices? And before anyone else?

What about awesome giveaways, amazing health tips and motivation? If that is something you are interested in, please visit the link below to join our newsletter:

www.HolisticWellnessBooks.com/newsletter

It's 100% free + spam free and you can easily unsubscribe whenever you want (although 99.9% of our readers decide to stay signed up and they love the book discounts and inspiration they are getting). We promise we will only email you with valuable and relevant information.

Oh, and as soon as you sign up, you will receive free instant access to an exclusive edition of our book *Alkaline Paleo Superfoods* to help you on your journey (and keep you reading until our next book is out!)

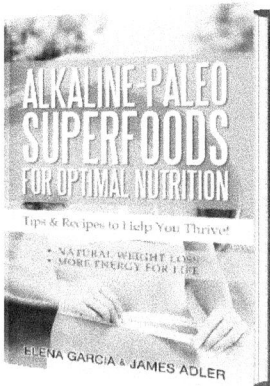

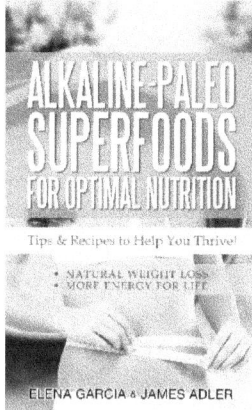

Sign up link: HolisticWellnessBooks.com/newsletter

*(note- please **DO NOT** sign up if you are **NOT INTERESTED** in getting email updates from us; we do not want to waste your time or disappoint you).*

More Books in the Paleo – Healthy Lifestyle Series

These books are available on Amazon in eBook, paperback and audiobook format.

You will find them by looking for *Elena Garcia* in your local Amazon store, or

Visiting:

HolisticWellnessBooks.com/elena

If you are in the UK, please visit:

HolisticWellnessBooks.com/elena-uk

Thank you again for taking an interest in my work,

Have an amazing day,

Elena

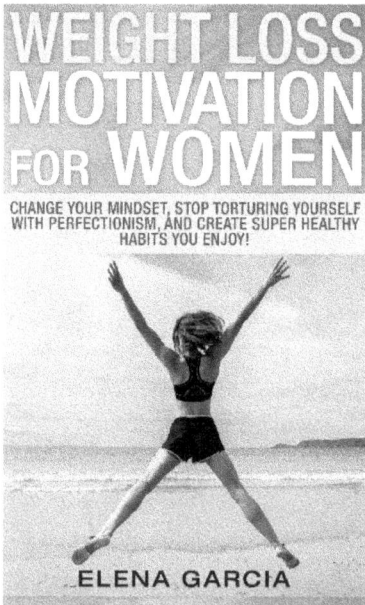

WEIGHT LOSS MOTIVATION FOR WOMEN

CHANGE YOUR MINDSET, STOP TORTURING YOURSELF WITH PERFECTIONISM, AND CREATE SUPER HEALTHY HABITS YOU ENJOY!

ELENA GARCIA

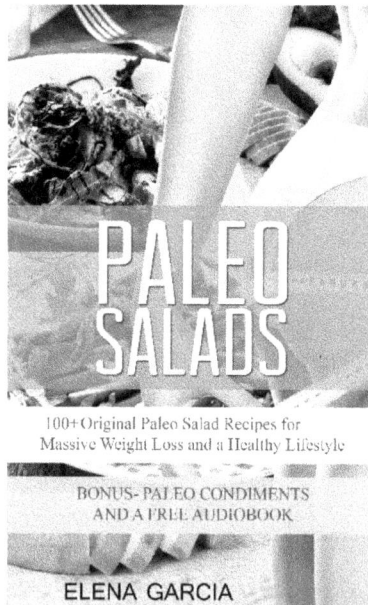

PALEO SALADS

100+ Original Paleo Salad Recipes for Massive Weight Loss and a Healthy Lifestyle

BONUS- PALEO CONDIMENTS AND A FREE AUDIOBOOK

ELENA GARCIA